About the booklet:

This booklet provides information on Fetal Alcohol Syndrome (FAS) and Fetal Alcohol Effects (FAE) to help support professionals in their work with clients whose lives have been affected by fetal alcohol exposure. Rather than simply describing the symptoms and tragedy of FAS/FAE, this booklet presents a framework for understanding the daily challenges faced by people with FAS/FAE and provides guidelines for educating clients about FAS and FAE. It also discusses strategies for working with these clients, beginning with identifying and understanding the source of their difficulties.

About the author:

Diane Malbin is a clinical social worker and cofounder of the Fetal Alcohol Syndrome/Drug Effects Clinical Programs in Portland, Oregon. Her background includes training in education and chemical dependency as well as social work. Her work focuses on proactive approaches to living and working with individuals who have Fetal Alcohol Syndrome (FAS) or Fetal Alcohol Effects (FAE), understanding the existing barriers to identification, and developing concrete, specific strategies for dealing with the problems of FAS and FAE. As a recovering alcoholic and birth parent of a child with FAE, she brings a personal component to her work.

Diane Malbin, M.S.W.

Fetal Alcohol Syndrome And Fetal Alcohol Effects

Strategies for Professionals

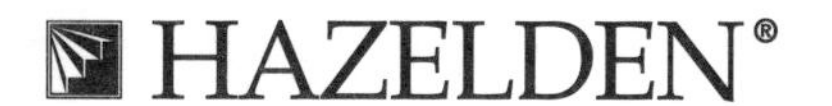
HAZELDEN®

Hazelden
Center City, Minnesota 55012-0176

ISBN: 0-89486-951-5

Introduction

Fetal Alcohol Syndrome (FAS), Fetal Alcohol Effects (FAE): What thoughts or feelings first come to mind as you read these words?

For many, these words evoke images of people who are isolated, hyperactive, aggressive, or high-school dropouts. When asked to describe images of where people with FAS or FAE might end up, many envision a future of hopelessness: in jail, on the streets, in institutions, as prostitutes, as alcoholics. These negative images come from newspaper articles, television specials, magazines, and books. Very few examples of positive outcomes have been portrayed in the mass media.

A very different picture of people with FAS/FAE is now emerging, however—one of hope and potential. Parents, teachers, and clinicians who have had direct and successful experiences working with people who have FAS or FAE use a different set of words to describe these people: loving, compassionate, artistic, determined, and hopeful.

The following people I know have at least one thing in common—they all have FAS or FAE: Ph.D. candidates, administrators, counselors, teachers, computer technicians and programmers, musicians, an electrician, a gardener, clients in recovery, and my daughter, who at thirteen is loving, caring, and determined. All of these people are successful in their personal and professional lives, and all have had struggles. But who of us hasn't?

Although the damaging effects of FAS and FAE are very real, there is increasing evidence, through personal stories and preliminary clinical findings, that with identification and supportive intervention, people with FAS/FAE are living healthy, successful lives. Professionals, parents, and people with FAS/FAE who understand their condition and are working to develop strategies that fit their individual needs are all making a difference.

What is the key for success? In a word: *identification.* Early identification supported by appropriate parenting, treatment, and educational strategies is optimal; identification at any point is pivotal for supporting people with FAS/FAE. But identification alone is not enough. To achieve long-term, comprehensive solutions we need to share information about FAS and FAE on a community-wide basis and among a range of disciplines. Chemical dependency professionals and other health care providers are in key positions to understand, identify, and provide support for people with FAS/FAE and their families.

This booklet provides chemical dependency counselors and others with information about FAS and FAE and presents a framework for understanding the physical and emotional effects. It also provides guidelines for educating clients about FAS and FAE and developing effective strategies for working with clients who have FAS or FAE. It does not, however, offer any promises or a recipe for success; the variability of effects is too great for a set approach.

My story

I am a recovering alcoholic. A little over thirteen years ago, I was a chronic late-stage alcoholic, living on welfare, a single parent with two small children. Since completing inpatient treatment, however, I have maintained sobriety, earned a graduate degree, and worked as a chemical dependency counselor. I currently work as a clinician, lecturer, and consultant.

My recovery story is not unique. We all have remarkable stories about our recoveries. What was new for me was discovering, midway through my graduate program in social work, three simple words. I heard them in class one evening, casually strung together in an earth-shattering way: *Fetal Alcohol Syndrome.* I was shocked. I'd never heard of FAS before. I had completed treatment and aftercare, gone to many meetings, and read about early childhood development, parenting in recovery, and children of alcoholics. I had even asked my children's pediatrician about possible effects, yet I had never heard or seen a single mention of "fetal alcohol" anything. I was stunned to discover later over two thousand articles had been written on FAS by the time my daughter was born.

After hearing the words "Fetal Alcohol Syndrome," I decided to face my fears directly: I would either put them to rest or learn what effects my drinking might have had. I read article after article on the effects of alcohol on children. The shock, denial, and grief that came with the dawning realization that my addiction had physically harmed my children were unutterable.

Although there is more public awareness about drinking and pregnancy today, many people still have little information about the effects of alcohol on children. I know from personal experience, from talking with people across the country and in Canada, that in every audience where people hear information about FAS and particularly FAE for the first time, some begin to identify their own children as having effects. FAE is common.

Many of us become chemical dependency professionals after addressing our own experiences with addiction and recovery. This includes recovery from growing up with alcoholic parents. Most of us in recovery hear about fetal alcohol or drug exposure the same way the rest of the country hears about it—in the media. Or we might hear about it at conferences. It is a shattering experience to read information as professionals—for our clients—only to discover we are reading for ourselves, for our own children, and for our friends' children.

This booklet is designed to support you in your work with clients as you provide them with information about FAS and FAE. The first and most important step in that process is supporting yourself. Should you identify your husband, wife, son, daughter, or even yourself as having FAE, know you're not alone. This is incredibly common. Find someone safe to talk with, and gather further information. Write or call the resources listed on pages 41-43. The resolution of this kind of grief eventually empowers us as professionals to rechannel the energy born of the grief into proactive works. The personal work comes first.

Fetal Alcohol Syndrome (FAS)

Fetal Alcohol Syndrome is now believed to be the leading cause of mental retardation in the Western world, and the only preventable one (Clarren 1992).

FAS is a medical diagnosis which has a very narrow set of diagnostic criteria. Physicians who first identified this pattern of malformations wanted to be sure that no other *teratogen* (a substance which causes changes in normal fetal development) could cause this condition.

There are thousands of possible teratogens. Fifty-three have been identified as having measurable effects. They include cigarettes, anticonvulsants (such as Dilantin), Valium, librium, and barbiturates, as well as other commonly abused substances, such as marijuana, cocaine, heroin, methadone, phencyclidine (PCP), and various designer drugs. The effects these substances have on infants include low birthweight, premature birth, labor problems, withdrawal symptoms, poor bonding, prenatal strokes, problems with vision and muscle tone, developmental delays, and cleft palates, among others.

This booklet focuses specifically on the effects alcohol has on children, for a few reasons. Recent research shows that the long-term effects of alcohol on fetuses are more powerful than those of other drugs, including cocaine (Chasnoff 1991). Also, most individuals use more than one substance if they use illegal drugs, and alcohol is often the second drug of choice. In one study of 250 women whose primary drug of choice was cocaine, only two did not also use alcohol to mitigate the effects of the cocaine (Streissguth, personal communication, 1993). Alcohol is the most used and abused drug in the world.

The Fetal Alcohol Study Group of the Research Society on Alcoholism standardized the definition of Fetal Alcohol Syndrome in 1980. Drs. Robert Sokol and Sterling Clarren proposed the following criteria in 1989:

1. Prenatal and/or postnatal growth retardation, where weight and/or length are below the tenth percentile when corrected for gestational age.

2. Evidence of central nervous system involvement: microcephaly (small head), tremulousness, poor coordination, learning disabilities, developmental delays, mental retardation, and behavioral dysfunction, including hyperactivity, among other symptoms.
3. A characteristic pattern of facial features and other physical abnormalities, including short palpebral fissures (eye openings), short upturned nose, low nasal bridge, flat philtrum (vertical groove between upper lip and nose), thin upper lip, and simply formed external ears, among others.

In order to be diagnosed as having FAS, a person must have at least one characteristic in each of these three categories. Having such a narrow diagnosis is a double-edged sword: It provides a clear picture of people with FAS, which leads to good research and interventions, but it also leaves most people whose mothers drank during pregnancy without a diagnosis.

Diagnosis is further complicated for many reasons. For example, the medical histories of the mothers are often unavailable, because frequently these children have been removed from their birth mothers before they are diagnosed as having FAS. In one study, only 3 percent of the children with FAS remained with their birth mothers (Streissguth, LaDue, and Randels 1988).

Paternal effects: effects on sperm and measurable outcomes on children

Fetal alcohol exposure is not just a women's issue; it never has been. Many women need support from their partners and extended family members in order to remain abstinent during pregnancy, but it goes further than that. What if a father's use of alcohol and other drugs also has measurable effects on his children? Right now we don't know definitively.

Many of the research findings we now have are based on animal studies; yet if even a portion of the findings are relevant to people, this research deserves careful attention.

The following possible effects have been documented in research, but it should be noted that some of the research is contradictory. Not all findings are uniformly supported by all researchers:

- In one study done on rats, paternal alcohol consumption resulted in decreased litter size, decreased testosterone levels in male offspring, and learning differences (Abel 1989).
- In a study on mice, paternal alcohol exposure resulted in offspring with decreased activity and decreased testosterone levels (Abel and Lee 1988).
- Research has found long-term changes and deficits in normal developmental and behavioral patterns spanning several generations, suggesting that male offspring may be more vulnerable to alcohol-induced alterations from fathers who consumed alcohol. Although this is from an animal study, researchers have concluded that the results may correlate with neurophysiological deficits among sons of human alcoholic fathers (Friedler 1987).
- Studies have shown that cocaine affects sperm structure and that this could result in abnormal development of the offspring of cocaine-exposed males (Yazigi, Odem, and Polakoski 1991; el-Gothamy and el-Samahy 1992).

Fetal Alcohol Effects (FAE)

Currently between one and three out of one thousand children in the general population are estimated to have FAS. However, 16 percent of the general obstetric population drinks enough during pregnancy to be at risk for producing children with some effects (NCADD 1990). Although there are no specific diagnostic criteria for Fetal Alcohol Effects, the following is an excellent working definition:

> A child with a history of prenatal alcohol exposure but not all the physical or behavioral symptoms of FAS may be categorized as having Fetal Alcohol Effects (FAE). *It should be noted that FAE is not the less severe form of*

Researchers are beginning to caution against causing undue anxiety in women and families. Since most women drink and most don't plan their pregnancies, women who drank prior to knowledge of being pregnant have expressed tremendous fear. It is important for them to know that the outcome for the baby is improved any time a woman stops drinking during pregnancy.

Pregnant women who have information about the possible effects of drinking on their babies and who *appear* to choose to continue to drink have probably lost the ability to choose. Denial, which is heard as rationalizing, may be an attempt to develop congruence between behaviors that are a function of compulsion and the woman's "knowing" she should not be drinking. Recognizing and addressing denial is essential. Telling her to "Just say no" doesn't work. The level of intervention needs to reflect the degree of deterioration and the nature of the denial in order to be effective.

Chemical dependency professionals are in a unique position in the wider professional community. Unlike many of their peers, they are not schooled to have absolute answers, given the nature of the disease process with which they work. The ability to tolerate ambiguity and view identification and intervention as processes is a valuable asset in working with people with FAS and FAE.

Characteristics associated with Fetal Alcohol Effects

A person who is mentally retarded may have trouble in all cognitive areas: learning new information, linking new information with old, remembering and recalling, doing something with what was learned. People with FAS/FAE, however, are often not affected across the board. They may have remarkable strengths in some areas and holes in others.

Their performance is often spotty. Some days they may be able to learn and follow through; other days they can't. It's terrifying for people not to be able to rely on their brains to perform consistently from day to day. Also, parents and professionals receive random reinforcement. The "on" days simply bolster our impression that the child is uniformly bright and capable, reinforcing the belief that the child could achieve if only he or she tried harder. This makes the "off" days especially important to understand.

The following information will help you understand what may seem like odd, bizarre, and inconsistent behavior. Understanding will also make clear the great frustration felt by people with FAS/FAE. People with FAS/FAE may provide the most invaluable insights into their experiences. Consider the following cases:

- One adult woman with FAE described how she has to "memorize life" in order to succeed. And succeed she has, as a professional and an administrator.
- One adult male described himself as "the man with a mind like a steel sieve." Another described his brain as "Swiss cheese."
- One man said he felt like he was "in a room with doors leading off of it, and sometimes the doors were all closed."
- A middle school student drew a picture of himself in a jail cell, his arm extended beyond the bars. In his hand he held a broomstick that was stretched toward the key to his cell, which was hanging on the wall nearby. The boy said, "And the broomstick is just an inch too short. Happens all the time."

Understanding Thought Processes

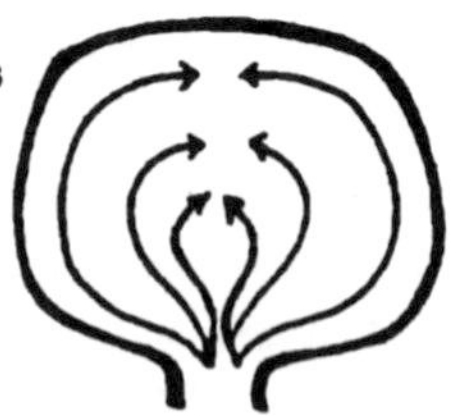

Normal development process: Orderly, organized, sequential. Many opportunities for links and interconnection.

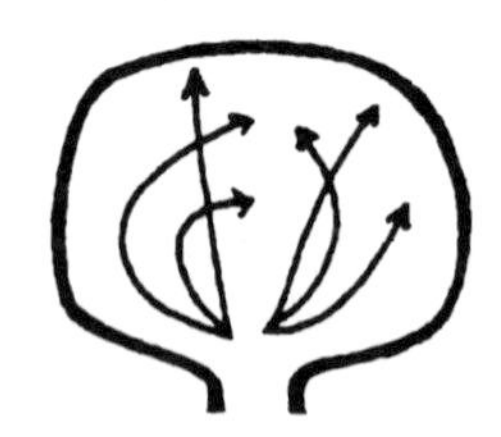

FAS/FAE: Inconsistent growth, undergrowth, overgrowth, disorganized gaps and clusters. Clusters can appear as areas of tremendous strength, such as superior ability in art, music, spelling, or writing.

Theoretical construct: making sense of the puzzle of FAS/FAE

Dr. Barbara Morse has developed a clear model for organizing and understanding the various confusing behaviors of people with FAS/FAE (1991). Her model, a variation on information-processing deficit models, isn't new, but how she addresses the academic and social behaviors of individuals with information-processing deficits *is* new. Before, when a child's area of weakness was discovered, parents and professionals pounced on it. People worked hard to bring that one area up to speed, whether it was math, reading, or memory. In other words, they tried harder to fix the deficit. That's a little like a mother trying every day for a full year to teach her son how to tie his shoelaces. It's a good intention, but it doesn't work. The key is to try differently rather than to try harder. Trying differently means the mother gets Velcro and tries with the shoelaces later.

In Dr. Morse's model, people with FAS and FAE often have trouble in three areas:

1. *Difficulty translating information from one sense or modality into appropriate behavior.* Translating hearing into doing, thinking into saying, reading into speaking, feelings into words.
2. *Difficulty generalizing information.* Links are not automatically formed. Learning happens in isolated clumps and may be unconnected or loosely connected to other experiences, thoughts, or emotions.
3. *Difficulty perceiving similarities and differences.* Without the ability to generalize and make associations, a person's capacity to compare and contrast, see whole patterns, sequence, predict, and judge is affected.

The above may be summed up in a single word: *gaps.*

Difficulty translating information from one sense into appropriate behavior: gaps in links

Difficulty linking what is heard with appropriate behavior

- People with FAS/FAE have been described as

"telephone answering machines." They may repeat word-for-word a simple request, and then go off and do something else, or forget halfway through a task what they were supposed to do. For example, a mother might say to her son, "Hang up your coat. What did I tell you?" "You said, 'Hang up your coat,'" the boy answers. He turns to go do the task, but slows down in the living room and stops to straighten some clutter. His mother walks in and says, "Thanks for doing the living room. Did you get your coat?" The boy shakes his head. "Please hang up your coat."

Able to "talk the talk, but not walk the walk."

- Their words and behaviors may not match.
- Their expressive language is often better than their receptive language; they speak better than they are able to comprehend. Their sheer amount of speech may mask shallowness of content or lack of connectedness with behavior.

Inconsistent mastery

- What's learned on Monday may be forgotten by Wednesday. They may get 100 percent on a test on one day, 25 percent on the same test a day later. Students affected by fetal alcohol exposure may need reteaching, more repetitions, or rechecking for actual comprehension.
- They may have difficulty mastering new skills and integrating these with earlier learning. They may be aware that they're not doing something right but can't figure out what it is.

Spotty memory

- Some memory functions are strong. For example, people with FAS/FAE may have a good long-term visual memory, but they may forget verbal instructions.
- People with FAS/FAE have been described as "computers" or "word processors" that get only part of what's needed on the screen. They need exactly the

be sincere about showing up next Monday at 2:00 P.M., but then they don't call and don't show.

- They learn better when they can touch, see, smell, hear, say, do.

Behavior that is socially inappropriate, intrusive

- People with FAS/FAE may miss social cues. Often these people are "in your face" or "in your space." The same behaviors that are cute when a person is five are seen as odd, inappropriate, and irritating when the person is sixteen. It's not uncommon to see a five-year-old drape herself over her mother's lap in public; it's disconcerting to see a sixteen-year-old do so. We have social expectations for appropriate behaviors at different ages. When there is a gap between our expectations and others' behaviors, we have problems.
- People with FAS/FAE may miss nonverbal cues. A parent was perplexed by his daughter's uncanny ability to accurately "read" how he was feeling. He said, "She reads me like a book, but when I give her a nonverbal cue about appropriate social behavior she doesn't get it!" The daughter could not apply the cue to her own behavior.

Additional symptoms that may indicate organic brain damage

While the above framework helps us organize and make sense of the various behaviors of people who have FAS/FAE, we also need to be aware of the following symptoms, which are associated with organic brain damage:

Distractibility

- May not filter out information received by all senses: hearing, sight, touch, smell, taste.
- May respond to all senses, all input, all the time. May not be able to prioritize which input is important or to filter out less important information.
- May be highly distractible, going from sound to sight to touch, eventually overloading on stimuli.

Irritability, excitability, or hyperactivity may develop. Unfortunately, most people with FAS/FAE don't have words to describe their experiences; they have no way of knowing that how they experience the world is different—not better or worse—than others.

Reactions to being overloaded vary from person to person. Some might become more excitable, more active. Others may "shut down" and withdraw, their faces blank and expressionless. Hours, days, months, even years later they may act out. Since the ability to form links between senses and behaviors, thoughts and speech may be impaired, the ability to put words on feelings may also be compromised. The feelings accumulate. Eventually people with FAS/FAE may begin to show a low threshold for frustration, blowing up over seemingly small events.

Slow cognitive pace

To complicate the picture, in addition to having hypersensitivity to stimuli, people with FAS/FAE may have a slow cognitive pace. It may take them longer to understand or act on what they are experiencing.

- *Hearing:* They may not immediately grasp the meaning of a word their ears just picked up. In normally paced conversation, it's as if they hear every third word. Unfortunately for them and those around them, they are often not able to say, "Please slow down." They typically try to look and act as if they understand. They want to look like everyone else, to fit in. With younger children, we may see increased acting-out behaviors when there is an invisible hearing deficit. Children may increase their physical activity, space out, utter off-the-wall comments, or talk with a friend.
- *Vision:* They may be able to decode words but not understand their meaning. Reading comprehension is frequently low. They may demonstrate dyspraxia, in which the hand doesn't seem to follow the brain's commands. (This may be related to sequencing problems.)

- *Speech:* Delays in cognitive processing may show up as long pauses between having a thought and expressing it or being asked a question and answering it. Gaps are often filled with "um's" or "ah's," or with off-the-wall comments, out-of-the-blue statements. They may overtalk to fill in the blanks.

For example, a teacher was explaining how to do a social studies problem to a student with FAS. The student didn't seem to get it, so the teacher did what most of us do when a person doesn't appear to understand: She expanded her explanation, tried harder, tried a few different ways to explain the concept to the boy. Finally, in frustration, he clamped his hands over his ears and said, "Shut up and talk to me!" At first the teacher was offended. After all, she was just trying to help. Then she got it; she understood he was overwhelmed by the sheer number of words he was hearing (Murphy 1991).

Perseveration

People with FAS/FAE often don't know when to let go, or quit. Children who have been exposed to alcohol and other drugs during pregnancy have been described as having difficulty making transitions from activity to activity, day to day, place to place. Sometimes they refuse, displaying anger and frustration when asked to go to the next task. This may reflect fears and discomfort that come from not knowing what's coming next. It may also reflect slow cognitive pace; it just takes them a little longer to finish a task. The urgency around needing to *finish* a task is intense.

Perseveration may relate to rigidity, which reflects their attempts to control and make sense of their environment. Because they have difficulty anticipating what will happen next, change may be frightening, and they may therefore resist it. When perseveration assumes the shape of repetitive self-stimulating behaviors, such as rocking or manipulating something in the hands, it may serve to form a pattern in an unpredictable world and soothe.

Hyperactivity
Eighty percent of all children identified as having FAS demonstrate hyperactivity. They often appear to outgrow it in adolescence. Many times the hyperactivity stems from overstimulation. Evaluating and modifying environments may significantly reduce hyperactive behaviors.

Although some children with FAS/FAE reportedly benefit from cautious medicinal interventions, others have either a paradoxical or idiosyncratic response to medications. In general, they are extremely sensitive to the effects of medications. A good guideline is to evaluate and modify environments first and to medicate as a last resort. It's important to recognize whether the decision to medicate is made more for the comfort of the parents or professionals or in the best interests of the child.

Tactile defensiveness
People with FAS/FAE may be extremely sensitive to light, sound, touch, taste, smell. Their skin may be so tender that rough seams on their clothing cause them pain. They may cut the bumps from the toe seams of their socks or wear clothes three sizes too large to avoid binding. Toothbrushing may hurt when bristles connect with gums. Conversely, some have been identified as hyposensitive to pain, and also to pleasure. There does seem to be a gradual modulation of both ends of the spectrum of hypo- to hypersensitivity over time.

Impulsivity
Other children may be better able to squelch their impulses to fidget. Children with FAS/FAE may simply show their discomforts more quickly and have less impulse control. When coupled with being easily distracted and unable to predict the consequences of behaviors, this impulsivity leads to many problems, especially when the child's behaviors are seen as willful.

The above behaviors are associated with organic brain differences. This is the most important thing for chemical

luxury of a clear and accurate history of maternal alcohol use during pregnancy. It's important to begin to look at patterns of behaviors. Begin to ask, "What if. . ."

Substance abuse professionals usually meet people with FAS/FAE and their family systems somewhere in the cycle of deterioration. It's challenging to try to unravel from a crisis which behaviors can be described as "acting out" because of family dysfunction and which indicate the presence of brain damage.

There are many diagnoses and descriptions of patterns of behaviors which overlap FAS/FAE. Typically, the symptoms identified in people with FAS/FAE cause them to be diagnosed with the following conditions rather than with FAS or FAE. These include

- Children or adult children of alcoholics (What population would also be most likely to have FAS/FAE?)
- Attention Deficit/Hyperactivity Disorder
- Attachment Disorder
- Sensory Integration Dysfunction
- Autism/Pervasive Developmental Disorders
- Oppositional Defiant Disorder

The above list is not exhaustive. The point is to show that people with FAS/FAE may have been identified in the past as hyperactive, attachment-disordered, or seriously emotionally disturbed. Not all people who are diagnosed with these conditions have FAS/FAE. However, given the current rates of underidentification of FAS/FAE, it is reasonable to assume that some *also have* FAS/FAE.

Any paradigm or diagnosis that fails to identify or incorporate the meaning of a degree of organic brain damage may in fact make matters worse. Good techniques which are diligently applied by parents and professionals and which work for some clients may not work with clients who have a degree of organic brain dysfunction. Parents, teachers, and clinicians often comment on how information about FAS/FAE is like the missing piece of a puzzle, one which pulls the pieces of the puzzle together and makes sense of it.

A normal human response to pain is to protect. As substance abuse counselors in particular well understand, defense systems develop as attempts to protect from pain. Over time, where there is cumulative pain, stress, and confusion, people with FAS/FAE (and those who live and work with them) develop defensive behaviors. Over more time, these behaviors may be reinforced and become rigid systems. In some cases they are identified as psychopathology. Traditional psychotherapy alone may end up confusing everyone and ultimately will blame the victim for "not trying."

Understanding the source of behaviors, not fixing symptoms

FAE is in a very real way an invisible handicapping condition. Alcohol compromises and modifies brain development and thus affects behaviors. One researcher has called it a "behavioral teratogen" (Morse 1991).

Dr. Sterling Clarren, walking through the library of the Centers for Disease Control, noted that in the section on handicapping conditions, the support literature presented strategies for modifying *environments* to help people with the various handicaps. When he came to the section on behaviors, however, he noted that the support literature in this section focused on changing *behaviors*. FAS/FAE is a physically handicapping condition; people with FAS/FAE learn differently, and their behaviors often indicate these differences. As for people with other handicaps, their environments need to be modified to support them (personal communication 1992).

The idea is to begin to think about how to modify environments. Environments may include attitudes, perceptions, physical layout, sensory stimuli, timelines, expectations, and processes. The goal is not to limit or enable people, nor is it to excuse or avoid. The goal is to support people in achieving appropriate behaviors and successes; the goal is to establish a win-win dynamic.

Traditional behavioral interventions are based on assumptions about abilities. Simply warning a person or giving a consequence for behaviors requires that he or she do the following cognitive gymnastics: link hearing with doing, compare and contrast, consider abstract options, generalize, and modify future behaviors based on the synthesis of the mental computations. What's wrong with this picture if the person has FAS or FAE?

Early identification of at-risk women and children has proven to yield good results at less cost—financial and emotional. Underidentification of at-risk parents and people with FAS/FAE is still the norm, however.

There are complex social, cultural, historical, and personal dynamics that play into the general discomfort around "naming" the variable—alcohol—especially when talking with women about drinking alcohol during pregnancy. These dynamics combine to severely impair prevention efforts and also have a direct impact on how chemical dependency and other professionals work with this issue. Currently, gaps in services and nonexistent resources in communities greet professionals seeking support for their work with people who have FAS/FAE. In spite of huge barriers to effectively identifying and supporting people with FAS/FAE, many people experience success and even help create resources in their communities.

Role of chemical dependency (CD) counselors in educating clients about FAS/FAE

Effectively addressing FAS/FAE presents an enormous challenge. Because of the complexity of the problem and the many ways in which people and families are affected, there's no one person, no one profession, and no one way to accomplish the task of prevention. When CD counselors are asked how they feel about providing clients with information on FAS/FAE, their first reaction is often frustration: "It's important but there's no room; there's no time. My day is already too full, length of treatment is being whittled down, and I have to make difficult decisions about which essential pieces to delete. There's already so much to know—I can't be an expert on everything. I can't do it *all*!"

Understanding personal and professional boundaries is

important. Since FAS is a medical diagnosis, CD counselors don't diagnose. But they are in key positions to provide information, educate, identify behaviors, intervene, support, and participate in a broad-based continuum of care. Developing aftercare links with other community members is vital for ongoing support. This is all part of prevention.

Addressing personal discomfort

It can be uncomfortable to talk with women about the effects of alcohol on developing babies—especially if their babies or they themselves have been affected.

Clinicians may avoid talking about FAS/FAE if they fear their clients will go away and never come back again, relapse, commit suicide, hate their parents, or adamantly deny they or their children could be affected by FAS/FAE. In short, a lot of catastrophizing happens.

Clinicians who would prefer to avoid addressing FAS/FAE offer many forms of denial: minimizing, rationalizing, "protecting." If the impetus for the denial is to protect the clinician from discomfort, that's important to know. Reducing that discomfort is important in order that it not be communicated to clients.

Discomfort is normal. Maybe a workable goal is not total elimination of all discomfort, but an acceptance, understanding, and reduction of it.

Introducing information about FAS/FAE: a process

There are probably as many viable, effective ways to begin to identify and explore FAS/FAE as there are skilled, knowledgeable, and caring clinicians.

First, it's okay not to know everything or have all the answers. In this field there are few experts. Gather information, and understand that this information is not tangential, it is pivotal. FAS represents the threshold of departure from the traditional paradigm of behavioral intervention. Professionals cannot just read the material, thinking "Oh! This is interesting. It explains a lot!" and then set it aside and go on with familiar methods of working with behaviors. The information is essential, foundational to developing appropriate strategies and providing effective help. Ignoring it will only worsen the situation. Here are some suggestions for beginning to take action:

1. *Know yourself.* Identify and discuss your beliefs, biases and barriers—personal and professional. Most people may experience anger, fear, or awkwardness when discussing this information with clients. Discomfort is normal; there is no shame or blame in recognizing and addressing discomfort. Role-playing the discussion with a colleague may be helpful.
2. *Know your own limits.* It is the ethical responsibility of clinicians not only to educate themselves about FAS/FAE, but also to get help from outside sources when they need it.
3. *Have a plan.* Evaluate your community and your agency for resources to provide a continuum of care. Identify key people you can refer clients to as appropriate. Maintain an updated file of referrals, with names, numbers, and specific details.
4. *Be clear about the benefits of providing this information to clients.* The potential for positive outcomes may range from supporting recovery, to preventing more FAS/FAE births, to intervening in the cycle of deterioration for children, thus reducing confusion, offering hope, and developing appropriate treatment and aftercare plans for people with FAS/FAE.
5. *Establish rapport.* This may require more than one interaction. Start by letting clients know how common FAS/FAE is and that personal identification is usual in all groups. Let them know that if they have some concerns or would like more information, they can talk with counselors who can also help them make connections outside of treatment. When addressing a group of people, it is important to let them know that they can talk to someone individually.

6. *Provide a context for the information.* "Most people drink, and few people plan their pregnancies. We're finding that with accurate identification there's help and hope." Normalize the conversation: "I talk with everyone about this." And do so.
7. *Remember, introduction of information about FAS/FAE is a process.* Gain a sense of what parents believe about outcomes for individuals with FAS/FAE. Provide additional information as appropriate.
8. *Be aware that some of your clients—adolescents and adults—may have FAS/FAE.* You will eventually need to refer them to aftercare resources for further help in identifying their problems, but while they are in your care you can gather information about early school performance, social experiences, or particular difficulties. Ask parents or siblings for examples of behaviors that were odd or perplexing. Look for cues, such as impulsivity, "manipulating," anger outbursts, school failure, money problems. Provide concrete vignettes that show normal patterns of behavior for people with FAS/FAE. Invite clients to share stories of their own experiences with perplexing or confusing behaviors or episodes of spotty memory. This may take time.
9. *When you speak with clients who think their drinking may have harmed their child or children, help them address their grief and resolve their guilt.* Many mothers have internalized the negative cultural images of women alcoholics and hide from the social stigmatization. There may be no greater pain in recovery than that associated with recognizing FAS/FAE. The grieving process is often complicated by the internalized shame. Mothers often expect and receive little support. It helps to provide clients with names of other birth mothers who have reached a place in their own recovery where they can provide support to others. Refer clients to appropriate grief and FAS/FAE parenting groups.

10. *With your client, develop a plan for continuity.* Together, figure out the next steps, the date and time for your next meeting, and whom to invite. Follow through.

Working with clients who have been identified as having FAS/FAE

During a weekly staff meeting on a residential treatment unit, one CD counselor presented her case: "John has been on the unit for two weeks. He behaves inappropriately with his peers and fails to comply with unit expectations, although he is superficially friendly, engaging, and compliant. His Step work shows he has little insight into his drinking and using; in fact, he's had to do all the objectives from his first treatment problem over again. In group he deflects constantly, goes off the subject, and appears to be in denial. When confronted he looks blank. He doesn't follow through. I think he's conning." Staff decided he was inappropriate for treatment and discharged him with the recommendation that he attend ninety AA meetings in ninety days, get a sponsor, and seek counseling for his Adult Children of Alcoholics (ACOA) issues.

Although this sounds like many clients, John happens to have FAE. Identifying the special needs of FAS/FAE clients on admission or during intake interviews may help foster staff understanding of some of the "resistant" behaviors and support the development of appropriate treatment plans. If you don't already have this information, gather information about history of grandparents' and parents' drinking patterns, time of onset, and significant events associated with drinking.

Because of the wide variability in the degree of effects and how people are affected, there's no one approach to working with this population. When challenged by a client, ask "What if. . ." and try differently rather than harder. There are some general guidelines, however, which help clarify areas of difficulty and support the development of strategies for working with clients who have FAS/FAE:

1. *Obtain a history.* Sometimes that means touching base with a variety of social service agencies that have already collected important information on your client. In the case of adoption where records are sealed or lost or in cases where mothers are deceased or in denial, begin to gather information. Is there a history of early school failure? Do behaviors combine to form a familiar pattern in his or her life?
2. *Observe patterns of behaviors.* Look for congruence between what they hear and how they follow through, or what they say and how they behave. Listen for echolalic speech (repetition of what others say) or flat affect (where events are simply reported). Keep "clean" anecdotal records, avoiding use of interpretive or judgmental words, such as "intentionally," "bright," or "manipulative."
3. *Keep treatment plans simple and concrete.* Use role-playing, storytelling, art, relaxation. Ask open-ended questions and look for long-term visual memory cues. Questions such as "Can you tell me about . . ." or "Can you show me . . ." or "What does that make you want to do?" all work better than "Why?"
4. *Integrate an awareness of an organic problem into work with clients.* A person who has difficulty with abstraction may not be able to identify and talk about feelings, for example. Putting words on emotions is challenging for many of us; for people with FAS/FAE it's especially abstract.
5. *Provide structure, not control.* Control tends to be top-down and sets up power struggles. Many strategies for problem-solving are other-initiated and therefore functionally irrelevant, usually failing to support individual empowerment and responsibility. Environments that are characterized by structure rather than control invite individuals to participate in clarifying their needs and developing appropriate strategies. They respect the individual, value his or

her strengths, and are more likely to elicit cooperation. Such an environment is especially appropriate for people with FAS/FAE, since they are most likely to be knowledgeable about their needs and learning strengths. Furthermore, their participation in developing strategies is more likely to affix tasks in memory, lead to accurate recall, and further reinforce their success and empowerment.

6. *Use strengths and interests to teach.* Often people with FAS/FAE have strong creative intelligence. Use music, art, a love of animals, or writing to support the treatment process. Remember that long-term visual memory may be clear.
7. *Identify cues for shut-down or agitation.* Validate their experiences and frustrations. Reduce their sense of extreme isolation by listening to them and acknowledging their struggles. Recognize and help identify physical cues as possible sources of discomfort; for example, hypersensitivity or overstimulation. Acceptance is a vital starting point.
8. *Use a buddy system as appropriate.* Have the buddy model appropriate behaviors, read with them, and explore their treatment questions.
9. *Keep It Super Simple.* One or two objectives, simply written, will be more effective than a more complicated plan. The behaviors that reflect the presence of FAS/FAE may actually be beneficial for recovery. Persistence, rigidity, determination, and simplicity, if tapped, are elements for sustained recovery.
10. *Reinforce unit or group expectations concretely.* Often clients with FAS/FAE talk nonstop. They may interrupt in group and monopolize conversation. A "talking stick," an object passed to the person whose turn it is to speak, may provide a concrete visual cue to help remind them to take turns. Listen for the nugget in their conversation. The initial quantity of speech often thins, allowing a key theme to emerge a bit at a time.
11. *Invite your clients to participate in the development*

of strategies that might work. A schedule handwritten by clients for turning in assignments, an art journal, or another creative technique that taps into their strengths are a few suggestions. To check for comprehension of expectations, ask clients to walk you through the unit or agency rules and expectations, demonstrating behaviors if possible. Recheck for retention of information and provide consistency.

12. *Walk clients through transitions.* Talk about the flow of the day, how things happen. Keep your words few. Double-check periodically to support learning, especially where there's random retrieval and retention.
13. *As discharge approaches, take clients to meetings near their home.* Try to integrate treatment and aftercare into their lives. Link them with a home group rather than giving them the responsibility for choosing one. Establish a network of AA sponsors willing to gain knowledge about FAS/FAE and to take a more active role in the sponsoring relationship to support the early recovery of your clients' special needs. People with FAS/FAE are suggestible, impulsive, and often unable to predict outcomes or consequences of behaviors. Yet they want to appear to be the same as their friends, so linking them with sober supports, practicing refusal skills, and having a plan are especially important for them.

Aftercare

A few resources to explore include the following:

- Recovery community
- Knowledgeable physicians, nurses, and other health care professionals
- Family systems therapists, art therapists, psychologists, counselors
- Case managers, social services resources
- Probation or parole officers, legal system

- Educators, vocational habilitation, job training resources
- Leisure and recreational resources
- Speech, language, vision, and hearing specialists
- Family, friends, advocates
- Structured living resources
- Employers

This list is not complete. There are many other professions and resources within communities that together can provide an ideal continuum of care to support clients, their family systems, and our professional work.

It is important, however, for professionals to have a realistic sense of services that actually exist. Reports from across the country indicate that gaps in services are commonly encountered. Interest in FAS/FAE is a grass-roots movement. Each of us is in a position to create more resources by providing information to receptive community members who can participate in a continuum of care. Develop a list of questions for potential resources and find out what resources are available to you.

In Fort Simpson, Northwest Territories, a wise woman spoke of her community. She said, "In our village we have had workshops on cultural loss and grief. We have had seminars on emotional, sexual, and physical abuse. Our conferences have dealt with alcoholism and ACOA issues. There is a saying that a community doesn't heal until the last trauma surfaces. I don't know if there are any other traumas out there. I don't think there can *be* any other traumas out there. This one, FAS/FAE, is our future."

Our children represent our hope and our future. Without them, we have no future. We need to go beyond what history never taught us: that to punish illness, to regulate and legislate in an attempt to control and contain, has never worked. We hope, for the sake of all of our futures, that we are moving toward enlightenment and knowledge.

References

Abel, E. L. 1989. Paternal and maternal alcohol consumption: Effects on offspring in two strains of rats. *Alcoholism* 13(4):533-41.

Abel, E. L., and J. A. Lee. 1988. Paternal alcohol exposure affects offspring behavior but not body or organ weights in mice. *Alcoholism: Clinical and Experimental Research* 12(3):349-55.

Biermeister, Richard. 1992. Parent Panel. Northwest Alaskan FAS/FAE Conference, October 6-8, Nome, Alaska.

Burgess Donna, and Ann P. Streissguth. 1990. Educating students with FAS/FAE. *Pennsylvania Reporter* 22(1):2211.

Chasnoff, Ira. 1991. Plenary Session. National Association for Perinatal Addiction Research and Education Conference, December 14-16, Chicago.

Clarren, Sterling K. 1992. Current understandings of FAS and FAE. Paper presented at conference, FAS and FAE Creating Community Solutions, October, Traverse City, Mich.

Friedler, Gladys. 1987. Effects on future generations of paternal exposure to alcohol and other drugs. *Alcohol Health and Research World* 12(2):126-29.

el-Gothamy, Z., and M. el-Samahy. 1992. Ultrastructure sperm defects in addicts. *Fertility and Sterility* 57(3):699-702.

Langendorfer, Sharon. 1992. Lecture. Denver Public Schools, April 25, Denver, Colo.

Malbin, Diane, and Antonia Rathbun. 1991. Notes developed as part of training materials called Fetal Alcohol Syndrome/Drug Effects Clinical Programs.

Morse, Barbara. 1991. Information processing: A conceptual approach to understanding the behavioral disorders of fetal alcohol syndrome," Paper presented at the First International Conference on Educating Students with FAS/FAE, February 8-9, Fairbanks, Alaska.

Murphy, Maureen. 1991. Hippety-hop velcroed to the floor. Paper presented at the First International

Conference on Educating Students with FAS/FAE, February 8-9, Fairbanks, Alaska.

NCADD (National Council on Alcoholism and Drug Dependence). 1990. *Fact Sheet.* New York: National Council on Alcoholism and Drug Dependence.

Sokol, Robert J., and Sterling K. Clarren. 1989. Guidelines for use of terminology describing the impact of prenatal alcohol on the offspring. *Alcoholism: Clinical and Experimental Research* 13(4):597-98.

Streissguth, Ann P. 1988. *Alcohol and Child/Family Health: A Conference with Particular Reference to the Preventions of Alcohol-Related Birth Defects,* ed. Geoffrey Robinson and Robert Armstrong. Vancouver, B.C.

Streissguth, Ann P., Helen M. Barr, and Paul D. Sampson. 1990. Moderate prenatal alcohol exposure: Effects on child IQ and learning problems at age 7 1/2 years. *Alcoholism: Clinical and Experimental Research* 14(5):662-69.

Streissguth, Ann P., Robin LaDue, and Sandra Randels. 1988. *A manual on adolescents and adults with Fetal Alcohol Syndrome with special reference to American Indians.* Indian Health Service Contract #240-83-0035 and 243-88-0166.

Yazigi, R. A., R. K. Odem, and K. L. Polakoski. 1991. Demonstration of specific binding of cocaine to human spermatozoa. *JAMA* 266(14):1956-59.

Resources

Organizations

Fetal Alcohol Syndrome Program, Department of Health
Maternal/Infant Health and Genetics
Sandra Randels, Coordinator
1704 N.E. 150th Street K17-8
Seattle, WA 98155-7226
Phone: (206) 368-4473

Fetal Alcohol Syndrome/Drug Effects Clinical Programs
Diane B. Malbin, M.S.W.
Antonia Rathbun, M.A.

9450 S.W. Barnes Road, Suite 220
Portland, OR 97225
Phone: (503) 292-2259

March of Dimes
1275 Mamaroneck Avenue
White Plains, NY 10605
Phone: (914) 428-7100

National Center for Education in Maternal and Child Health
38th and R Streets, NW
Washington, DC 20057
Phone: (202) 625-8400

National Organization on Fetal Alcohol Syndrome
1815 H Street, NW, Suite 750
Washington, DC 20006
Phone: 1-800-66 NOFAS
Phone: 1-800-666-6327

Office of Substance Abuse Prevention
5600 Fishers Lane
Rockville, MD 20857
Phone: (301) 443-0373

Newsletters

FAS and Other Drugs Update
Prevention Resource Center
822 South College Street
Springfield, IL 62704
Phone: (217) 525-3456

The Iceberg
P.O. Box 95597
Seattle, WA 98145-2597

Curricula

Preventing FAS Curricula
Association for Retarded Citizens
500 E. Border St., Suite 300
Arlington, TX 76010

Fetal Alcohol Syndrome Facts and Choices, A Guide for Teachers
Wisconsin Clearinghouse
University of Wisconsin
P.O. Box 1468
Madison, WI 53701-1468

Videos

What is FAS?
Perennial Education
930 Pitner Avenue
Evanston, IL 60202
Phone: 1-800-323-9084

One For My Baby
AIMS Media
6901 Woodley Avenue
Van Nuys, CA 91406-4878

Straight from the Heart
Vida Health Communications
6 Bigelow St.
Cambridge, MA 02139

Other titles you can use with your clients . . .

A Woman's Loss of Choice, A Child's Future
How Alcohol and Other Drug Use During Pregnancy Affect Our Children
by Jeanne Engelmann
An excellent resource for women who worry that their drinking during pregnancy may have affected their children. Written in an easy-to-read style, this illustrated booklet explains the basics of Fetal Alcohol Syndrome and Fetal Alcohol Effects. It also includes information on how chemical use may affect a child's development during pregnancy and provides facts on what to do and where to go for help if a child is alcohol- or drug-affected. 16 pp.
Order No. 5544
